# BLASTOMYCOSIS INFECTIOUS DISEASE

## Fungal Infections That Can Affect Both Humans and Animals

## Dr. Betty C. Redding

# TABLE OF CONTENT


INTRODUCTION

CHAPTER 1
WHAT IS MEANT BY THE TERM BLASTOMYCOSIS
Transmission
Possible blastomycosis symptoms
The Identification of Blastomycosis
Mycological cultures and smear examination
Treatment
Prevention

# CHAPTER 2

## DISSEMINATED BLASTOMYCOSIS


Extrapulmonary blastomycosis

The Osseous Blastomycosis

Central Nervous System blastomycosis (CNS)

Pathogenesis

Host Reaction

Clinical Manifestations

Blastomycosis in Those Who Have Weak Immune Systems (HIV/AID, Women Who Are Pregnant and Their Newborn Babies)

Hematogenous dissemination

Signs and Symptoms of Blastomycosis

# CHAPTER 3

## BLASTOMYCOSIS SKIN

Papulopustular lesions

Cutaneous lesions

Causes

# CHAPTER 4

## BLASTOMYCOSIS IN DOGS

Manifestations and Methods of Diagnosis

Diseases

Breeds That Are Affected

Treatment

The Expense of Veterinary Care

Prevention

# CHAPTER 5

THE BLASTOMYCES DERMATITIDIS
BACTERIUM
Infection caused by fungi in the
recipient of an organ transplant
Pulmonary Illness and Its Molecular
Foundations
Infectious Disorders of the Kidney
Endemic mycoses
Infections of the Central Nervous
System Caused by Yeasts and Molds
Diseases Caused by Mycobacteria,
Fungi, Spirochetal Organisms, and
Parasites
Fungal infections that have spread
via the bloodstream hematogenous


CONCLUSION

# INTRODUCTION

Blastomycosis is a systemic fungal infection that can affect both humans and animals. It is caused by a fungal organism called Blastomyces dermatitidis, which has two distinct forms. Inhalation of spores that have been formed by the filamentous phase of the fungus is what starts the infection process in motion.

This phase of the organism can be found in nature or the laboratory at a temperature of 25 degrees Celsius, and it can transform into the yeast phase when it reaches 37 degrees Celsius in the lungs of an infected host. The disease can cure itself, but it is also possible for the pulmonary tissue to be in an acute or chronic state.

If the condition is left untreated while it is present in the lungs, it has the potential to become invasive and spread to other organs, as well as the central nervous system, where it may cause deadly meningitis. Blastomycosis and other systemic mycoses are collectively referred to as "developing fungal dangers." This is because not only do they infect people with healthy immune systems, but they also pose a risk to people who already have compromised immune systems.

Blastomycosis is highly endemic in certain regions of the upper midwestern states, including parts of Wisconsin and Minnesota, and has been linked to the southeastern and south-central states that border the Ohio and Mississippi Rivers as well as the southeastern and south-central states that border the Ohio and Mississippi Rivers.

Researchers have begun to pay a greater amount of attention to the development of methods for identifying, preventing, and treating mycoses as a direct result of the rise in the prevalence of systemic fungal illnesses. To gain a deeper comprehension of the immunobiology of the organism, the primary focus of research that has been conducted in our laboratory throughout the past few years has been on the examination of numerous strains of B. dermatitidis obtained from a living thing, animal, or enviro specimens collected from a wide variety of geographic locations. The disease has been difficult to diagnose for several reasons.

Although culturing and histological investigation can be helpful in certain situations, it is possible that these approaches will not produce the results that are needed in other cases. This has increased the amount of research being done to improve immunological assays, which tend to provide a more rapid diagnosis. Despite this, we and many other investigators are aware that there are still issues regarding the sensitivity and specificity of immunoassays.

In the current studies that we are conducting, we are looking into various combinations of the different B. dermatitidis yeast lysate antigens to determine how well they detect antibodies in serum samples taken from dogs that have blastomycosis.

# CHAPTER 1
# WHAT IS MEANT BY THE
# TERM BLASTOMYCOSIS

Blastomycosis is an extremely uncommon fungal infection that is typically contracted by inhaling the spores of the fungus Blastomyces dermatitidis or Blastomyces Gilchrist.

These fungi are most likely to be discovered in the damp soils that are present in wooded regions and beside waterways. Those residing in Ontario, Manitoba, as well as the south-central, south-eastern, and mid-western regions of the United States, are the most likely to be affected by blastomycosis.

Blastomycosis is most prevalent in the counties located in the state's northeastern region, but cases have been documented all around Minnesota.

In addition to monitoring human patients with blastomycosis, the Minnesota Department of Health and the Board of Animal Health also track animal cases.

This allows us to better identify where in the state the sickness is concentrated. More animals than humans are diagnosed with the disease each year, and in many cases, the exact location where the animal was first exposed to the fungus can be determined.

## Transmission

As a result of being released from contaminated soil, spores can travel into the air and cause blastomycosis when inhaled. Spores are more likely to become airborne during activities like digging, building, and clearing forests that take place on polluted soil.

In highly unusual circumstances, the fungus can invade an open skin wound and cause an infection there only.

Blastomycosis cannot be spread from person to person or from animal to human.

Knowledge of the disease's epidemiological risks and geographic distribution is essential for including blastomycosis in the differential diagnosis of individuals with lung, cutaneous, bone, or central nervous system infections. The only regions in North America where Blastomyces could be found naturally are the midwestern, south-central, and southeastern United States, and four Canadian provinces extending from Saskatchewan to Quebec. Blastomyces do not have a consistent distribution throughout the endemic area; rather, it is found in forested areas, has sandy soils with antacid H, have decaying plant or organic waste, and have rotting wood near pools of water.

This ecological subsegment is typified by acidic, sandy soils rich in decomposing plant and animal matter and rotting timber. Like H. capsulatum and Cryptococcus, Blastomyces can flourish in bird guano.

Although most cases of the disease are isolated incidents, it has been linked to occupations and hobbies that cause soil disturbance, such as building, digging, exploring beaver dams or underground forts, using society compost stacks, trimming bushes or cutting trees, hunting, canoeing, boating, tubing, and fishing. Most human cases of this disease result from contact with diseased animals.

## Possible blastomycosis symptoms include the following:

- If you cough, you might as well bring up some blood.
- Fever
- Apprehensive, shallow breathing
- Having nocturnal sweats and/or chills Exhaustion
- Pain in the muscles, joints, or bones, leading to loss of appetite and weight
- Discomfort in the chest or the back
- Chronic skin wounds that refuse to close.

There's a significant amount of variation in the amount of time that passes between being exposed to the spores and the onset of symptoms, with the range being anything from 21 to 100 days.

There is a wide range of variability in the signs and symptoms of blastomycosis across different people. An estimated fifty percent of all infections are either asymptomatic (the person does not develop any symptoms or disease) or minor and resolve on their own without therapy.

Some people end up with a persistent lung infection, and the illness can also spread to other parts of the body (skin, bones, central nervous system, or genitourinary system).

How long someone has had their disease

The symptoms of blastomycosis can continue anywhere from a few weeks to several years, depending on the individamongual patient.

## The Identification of Blastomycosis as the Disease in Question

The following tests are  those that can be used to diagnose blastomycosis:

- Culture (Species of Blastomyces can be isolated from infected tissues such as skin, skin biopsies, respiratory samples, and lung biopsies.)

- Smear for cytological examination (direct microscopic identification of broad-based budding yeast)
- Histopathology of tissue samples obtained by surgical biopsies.
- Urine antigen test or serum antigen test
- Antibody screening using serum (less reliable)

To further assist in determining whether or not you may have been exposed to Blastomyces spores, your physician may inquire about your past travels, hobbies that involve spending time outside, or the surroundings of your home.

## Mycological cultures and smear examination

### *Blastomyces urine antigen*

If there is a reason to suspect blastomycosis, a chest X-ray should be performed. Infiltrates can be either focal or diffuse, and they can sometimes appear as patchy bronchopneumonia radiating out from the hilum. It is necessary to differentiate these findings from other potential causes of pneumonia (eg, other mycoses, tuberculosis [TB], tumors).

Lesions on the skin have the potential to be misdiagnosed as sporotrichosis, tuberculosis, iodism, or even basal cell cancer. The condition can be misdiagnosed as genital tuberculosis.

Cultivation of infected material has been completed, and when positive, the results are conclusive. Because growing Blastomyces in culture can present a significant risk of infection to the people working in the laboratory, the laboratory ought to be informed of the possible diagnosis.

During a microscopic inspection of tissues or sputum, the distinctive appearance of the organism, which can also be diagnostic, can sometimes be observed.

The serologic test is not sensitive but can be helpful if it comes up positive.

A urine antigen test can be helpful, although there is a high risk of cross-reactivity with Histoplasma.

There are validated molecular diagnostic procedures available for Blastomyces, such as the polymerase chain reaction (PCR).

As a result of the non-specific nature of the clinical presentation, physical exam, and radiographic symptoms of blastomycosis, a high index of suspicion is required for rapid diagnosis.

Even in locations where the disease is endemic, it is usual for there to be a delay in diagnosis because very few patients are accurately diagnosed upon their initial presentation, and delays in diagnosis lasting longer than one month can occur in more than forty percent of patients.

A thorough history that identifies potential exposures and hosts who are at risk can make it easier to make a diagnosis. In patients who have pneumonia, the medical history should include information about the patient's place of residence, travel, hobbies, recent house renovation, exposure to road building, and use of a wood-burning stove or community compost pile, among other things.

Blastomycosis in a household pet, such as a dog, implies that there is a common source of exposure and can serve as a precursor to the disease in humans. In individuals who are suffering from both pulmonary and cutaneous diseases at the same time, blastomycosis needs to be taken into consideration as a potential diagnosis.

## Diagnostic techniques based on microscopy and culture

Examining clinical specimens that have been stained continues to be the quickest approach to making a diagnosis of blastomycosis. Sputum or tissue samples stained with 10% potassium hydroxide, calcofluor white, Gomori methenamine silver (GMS), or periodic acid-Schiff (PAS) can facilitate visualization of the characteristic Blastomyces yeast. This is in contrast to the fact that Blastomyces are not well visualized with hematoxylin and eosin (H&E) stains.

Before the results of culture and non-culture tests are available, a presumptive diagnosis of blastomycosis can be made based solely on the observation of the characteristic yeast forms associated with blastomycosis, which range in size from 8 to 20 M and have broad-based budding and a doubly refractile cell wall.

In one case series, the identification of over 80% of cases that were later validated by culture was achieved by correctly staining clinical specimens.

Even though fungal-specific stains are an excellent diagnostic tool, this method is frequently neglected. In tissue specimens, the presence of neutrophilic infiltration with noncaseating granulomas (also known as pyogranulomatous inflammation) can be suggestive of blastomycosis; hence, a comprehensive microscopic investigation for Blastomyces yeast should be carried out.

The conclusive diagnosis can be obtained from the Blastomyces culture. When pulmonary blastomycosis is present, the yield of culture that can be obtained with invasive bronchoscopy is very high. According to the findings of one investigation, the diagnostic yield of bronchoscopy was 92%. Even noninvasive methods, such as growing Blastomyces from sputum, tracheal discharge, or gastric washings, resulted in the development of the fungus in 86% of the samples.

Growth requires the use of specialized media such as brain-heart infusion medium, potato dextrose agar, and Sabouraud dextrose agar. Temperatures in the incubator that range from 25°C to 30°C and are employed in the majority of clinical laboratories encourage the growth of Blastomyces as a mold.

In culture, Blastomyces grows quite slowly despite its highly specialized nature. It takes anywhere from five to fourteen days for fungal colonies to become visible on average; however, when the infection burden is low, growth might take far longer.

## Non-culture diagnostics

Due to low sensitivity and specificity, traditional antibody testing, such as complement fixation (CF) or immunodiffusion (ID), is not clinically effective for the diagnosis of blastomycosis.

The sensitivity (87%) and specificity (94–99%) of an updated enzyme immunoassay (EIA) that employs microplates coated with BAD1 protein have been improved; however, this EIA is not currently available for purchase on a commercial scale.

Histoplasmosis and blastomycosis can be distinguished from one another by using BAD1 tests because BAD1 is only found in Blastomyces.

CF and ID have been replaced by an antigen assay that can test urine, serum, BAL fluid, and CSF specimens for the presence of Blastomyces. This assay can also detect a galactomannan component that is present in the cell wall of Blastomyces.

Antigenuria has a sensitivity ranging from 76.3 to 92.9% in individuals who have a condition that has been established, while its specificity is 79.3%. In the presence of other fungal illnesses, such as histoplasmosis, paracoccidioidomycosis, or penicilliosis, it is possible for a test to produce a false positive result (talaromycosis).

The clinical consequence of a false positive test is frequently limited because penicilliosis and paracoccidioidomycosis can be excluded from the differential diagnosis if the patient has not traveled to Southeast Asia and China (paracoccidioidomycosis) or Central and South America (paracoccidioidomycosis) (talaromycosis).

In addition, the treatment for blastomycosis is quite comparable to the treatment for histoplasmosis. Monitoring a patient's reaction to treatment using serial urine antigen concentrations is a possibility.

After starting treatment, a patient may see an increase in antigenuria (after a median of 11 days), which is then followed by a gradual decrease in antigen titer if treatment was successful.

The initial post-treatment rise in titer may reflect increased urine excretion of antigens as a result of the death of fungal cells.

The Appearance of Things on Radiographs

There are no radiographic patterns that can be used to reliably diagnose pulmonary blastomycosis.

The abnormalities on the radiograph are vague and could be misinterpreted as bacterial pneumonia, TB, or even cancer. Diffuse airspace illness, consolidation, nodular masses, interstitial disease, cavitation, and military diseases are all examples of radiographic abnormalities.

Consolidation is the most prevalent finding on radiographs and can be visible even in the absence of other pulmonary symptoms. Rarely seen are calcified lung lesions, hilar/mediastinal adenopathy, and pleural effusions. MRI is the imaging modality of choice for diseases of the central nervous system and is usually abnormal in patients who have blastomycosis of the central nervous system.

# Treatment

- Anti-fungal medicine can be used to treat blastomycosis; however, treatment with these drugs must typically be maintained for at least one year.
- Antibiotics that were developed to treat bacterial infections are ineffective against blastomycosis.
- Your healthcare professional is the best person to answer any specific questions you may have regarding the treatment.
- Itraconazole is recommended for patients with mild to moderate illness. Amphotericin B is used in cases of severe, life-threatening illness.

(For more information, Antifungal Medications and the Practice Guidelines for the Treatment of Blastomycosis published by the Infectious Diseases Society of America.)

In patients who do not receive treatment, blastomycosis often worsens gradually and only rarely results in death. The severity of the illness should be evaluated before beginning treatment for blastomycosis.

Itraconazole is taken orally at a dose of 200 milligrams three times a day for three days, after which it is taken either once a day or twice a day for a period of six months to a year depending on the severity of the disease. It appears that fluconazole is less effective, although patients who are intolerant to itraconazole and have a moderate illness may benefit from trying 400 to 800 mg orally once a day.

- Intravenous amphotericin B is usually successful in treating serious infections that endanger a patient's life. According to the recommendations made by the Infectious Diseases Society of America, patients should take a lipid formulation of amphotericin B at a dosage of 3 to 5 mg/kg once a day or amphotericin B deoxycholate at 0.7 to 1.0 mg/kg once a day for 1 to 2 weeks or until an improvement in their condition is observed.

As patients show signs of improvement, the treatment is switched to oral itraconazole; the dosage is 200 mg three times a day for three days, and then 200 mg twice a day for at least a year.

Patients who have blastomycosis of the central nervous system, pregnant patients, and immunocompromised patients should be treated with intravenous amphotericin B (ideally liposomal amphotericin B), following the same dose schedule as for life-threatening infections.

Although voriconazole, isavuconazole, and posaconazole are effective against B. dermatitidis, there is a dearth of clinical data on these drugs, and it is not yet clear what role they should play in treatment.

## The vast majority of patients with blastomycosis will require antifungal treatment.

The majority of patients who have blastomycosis will require therapy with antifungal medicine that is prescribed by a doctor. Itraconazole is a type of antifungal medicine that is commonly utilized in the treatment of blastomycosis that has been categorized as mild to moderate.

In cases of severe blastomycosis in the lungs or infections that have spread to other parts of the body, amphotericin B is typically prescribed as the treatment of choice. The duration of treatment might be anything from six months to one year, depending on the severity of the illness and the person's immune state.

Recommendations for the diagnosis and treatment of blastomycosis have been issued by the American Thoracic Society and the Infectious Disease Society of America. The location and intensity of the illness, as well as the host's immune condition and whether or not the patient is pregnant, all factor into the treatment recommendations.

Treatment with an antifungal medication is strongly suggested for all patients who have been diagnosed with blastomycosis, including those whose clinical symptoms have resolved before beginning therapy.

Before beginning treatment, a baseline assessment of the patient's hematologic, hepatic, and renal functions should be performed.

It is necessary to conduct a thorough examination of all prescriptions to reduce the risk of adverse drug interactions, which are frequently caused by azole antifungals. Itraconazole, voriconazole, posaconazole, and fluconazole all have the potential to lengthen the QT interval, and this effect is exacerbated when these antifungal agents are used with other medicines that also have this effect. Isavuconazole, on the other hand, has been shown to reduce the QT interval, which makes it inappropriate for people who have familial short QT syndrome. Itraconazole has the potential to worsen existing congestive heart failure (CHF), and as a result, it should be used with extreme caution in patients who already suffer from ventricular dysfunction. It also has a negative inotropic effect.

Antifungals that contain azoles raise the serum concentration of HMG-CoA reductase inhibitors that are processed via cytochrome P450 3A4, which can enhance the risk for statin-induced rhabdomyolysis.

Because it is not metabolized by P450 3A4, pravastatin can be taken with azoles without fear of adverse effects. Medications used to suppress the immune system, calcium channel blockers derived from dihydropyridine, sulfonylureas, and anticonvulsants are examples of other notable drug-drug interactions involving azoles.

Because of the potentially harmful consequences that azole exposure can have on pregnancy, including teratogenicity, all females of reproductive age must undergo pregnancy testing.

Amphotericin B (AmB) Polyene AmB formulations are suggested for the treatment of patients who have a severe lung infection, disseminated disease, central nervous system involvement, and underlying immunosuppression (for example, HIV/AIDS or SOT).

In addition, AmB is the first-choice treatment for neonates and women who are pregnant. AmB deoxycholate has a proven history of therapeutic success, with high rates of overall patient recovery. Even though it is effective, the usage of amB is linked to a large amount of cumulative toxicity.

- Nephrotoxicity is the most typical treatment-limiting toxicity, and it affects more than thirty percent of patients who are being treated. Other adverse effects include infusion reactions (such as fever, rigors, hypoxia, nausea, vomiting, hypertension, or hypotension) and electrolyte disturbances. Other adverse effects include fever, rigors, hypoxia, nausea, vomiting, hypertension, or hypotension (hypokalemia, hypomagnesemia).

- Infusions of 0.9% normal saline should be given before and after AmB treatment to reduce the risk of nephrotoxicity. Additionally, the use of diuretics and other nephrotoxic agents should be avoided.

To compensate for the kidneys' loss of potassium and magnesium, the majority of patients need to take potassium and magnesium supplements regularly.

With amB therapy, it is vital to perform frequent monitoring of electrolytes and creatinine levels (e.g., at least 2–3 times per week). Because these formulations have lower rates of nephrotoxicity, lipid AmB preparations (such as liposomal amphotericin, AmB lipid complex, and AmB colloidal dispersion) are preferred over AmB deoxycholate. Other examples include liposomal amphotericin.

- Liposomal amphotericin is the polyene of choice for the treatment of CNS blastomycosis because, of all the lipid formulations, it is the one that can penetrate the blood-brain barrier the most effectively.
- Triazoles

In contrast to AmB, antifungal drugs belonging to the azole class are fungistatic when applied to Blastomyces.

Itraconazole is the drug of choice for treating mild to moderate non-CNS blastomycosis and for step-down therapy after induction treatment with amphotericin B. It is also the drug of choice for step-down therapy.

The oral formulation of itraconazole can be prescribed as either a solution or a capsule;

however, the administration of these two different formulations is not the same.

Because serum concentrations are influenced by formulation, dosage, and interpatient variability in drug metabolism, therapeutic drug monitoring (TDM) is essential for optimizing itraconazole dosing.

This is because serum concentrations are measured in milligrams per milliliter (mg/mL). When compared to the capsule formulation, the usage of the solution results in serum concentrations that are roughly thirty percent greater.

Itraconazole solution can be taken regardless of whether or not food is being consumed, and it does not require the presence of stomach acid to be absorbed. To achieve the best possible absorption, it is necessary to take itraconazole capsules in conjunction with meals and an acidic beverage.

As a result, the solution form of itraconazole is the one that should be used for treating individuals who are already taking H2-blockers or proton-pump inhibitors. After two weeks of treatment, when a steady state concentration has been attained, it is recommended that levels of itraconazole be measured.

It is irrelevant when the itraconazole dose was administered to obtain serum specimens for TDM because the long half-life of approximately 24 hours enables this. Serum specimens can be obtained at any time. The total itraconazole level is determined by summing the concentrations of itraconazole and hydroxy-itraconazole, with a target level that falls anywhere between 1 and 5.5 Hg/mL. Antifungal effects can be attributed to the metabolite hydroxy-itraconazole, which is formed from itraconazole.

It is not necessary to have serum levels lower than 10.0 ug/mL because doing so is associated with increased medication toxicity. Tests of liver function should be performed at the beginning of treatment, then again after 2 and 4 weeks, and then every three months after that.

Voriconazole, posaconazole, and isavuconazole are some of the more recent triazoles that are active against B. dermatitidis. To have the best possible absorption, voriconazole should be taken on an empty stomach. Voriconazole should have a trough concentration in the serum that is between 1 and 5.5 g/mL when it is optimally used. 80 Posaconazole solution is best absorbed by high-fat meals, whereas posaconazole delayed-release tablets are unaffected by either food or gastric acid inhibitors.

Posaconazole solution is best absorbed by high-fat meals.

Although the optimal concentration of posaconazole is not established, the vast majority of industry professionals advise maintaining a level that is larger than 0.5 to 1 g/mL.

Isavuconazole can be taken orally without concern for food or the amount of acid produced by the stomach, and there is no requirement for TDM. Parental forms are available for voriconazole, posaconazole, and isavuconazole.

Both voriconazole and posaconazole are effective treatments for blastomycosis, with voriconazole also being used to treat infections of the central nervous system.

## Both steroid use and ARDS

The fatality rate of blastomycosis-induced ARDS remains high despite the administration of effective antifungal medication. Case studies have hinted at the possibility that supplementary steroids could enhance survival; however, a recent retrospective investigation of 43 patients diagnosed with ARDS owing to blastomycosis between the years 1992 and 2014 did not demonstrate this possibility.

A decrease in the patient's overall death rate who were given steroids. However, a greater study is required to determine the optimal dose, duration, and efficacy of adjuvant steroids in patients with ARDS.

## *Mortality*

Case fatality rates between 4.3 and 6.3% have been reported in large case series from the states of Wisconsin and Manitoba.

Death has been linked to a shorter duration of symptoms, which most likely indicates a more severe presentation and a weakened immunological condition in the patient. Even among patients who are receiving the correct antifungal treatment, the mortality rate is significant in individuals who have ARDS caused by blastomycosis.

Among AIDS patients who have not had immune reconstitution, the mortality rate associated with blastomycosis is close to forty percent, and the majority of deaths take place within three weeks after diagnosis.

In a similar vein, the death rate of patients who have had their immune systems suppressed by solid organ transplantation ranges from 33–38%, and this number rises when respiratory failure is present.

# Prevention

Regrettably, there are currently no known effective preventative treatments for blastomycosis that may be used.

There is not currently a technology that can test the soil to determine whether or not Blastomyces species are present.

Early diagnosis and treatment of blastomycosis, when necessary, can significantly lessen the severity of the illness caused by this fungal infection.

Early detection of the disease requires not only general public awareness but also awareness on the part of medical professionals.

# CHAPTER 2
# DISSEMINATED
# BLASTOMYCOSIS

Disseminated Blastomycosis has spread beyond the lungs and throughout the body.

The Blastomyces fungus is capable of spreading to any organ in the body. In around 25 to 40 percent of cases, there will be evidence that the disease has spread.

## Extrapulmonary blastomycosis

Is considered a disseminated disease and should be treated as such.

The only exception to this rule is the extremely rare instances of direct inoculation that occur as a result of penetrating trauma, accidental needle stick, or laboratory exposure.

## The Osseous Blastomycosis

Bone is the second most common region for Blastomyces to spread to after the skin. Between 5 and 25% of patients experience this. A condition known as pulmonary blastomycosis is present in the majority of patients with osteomyelitis.

Osseous lesions might be accompanied by painful soft tissue abscesses, draining sinus tracts, or skin ulcers.

Radiographic findings such as lytic destruction, periosteal reaction, or sclerotic margins, and histopathological findings such as granulomatous inflammation, are diagnostic of

Blastomyces-induced osseous invasion. Infection can occur in any bone in the body, but it most commonly affects the long bones, vertebrae, skull, and ribs. Bone mycosis, also known as blastomycosis, can mimic other diseases, including sarcoma, giant cell tumors, and even metastases (Mycobacterium tuberculosis).

Bone infections often result in septic arthritis or abscesses when they spread to neighboring joints or soft tissue. The term "direct extension" describes this method. Bone deterioration over time might cause a pathologic fracture (e.g. vertebral body collapse).

There was an estimated 20-30% GU spread in the case of a series with genitourinary blastomycosis published in the 1950s. However, less than 10% of individuals in the recent case series had prostate involvement.

The prostate and epididymis are the most common sites of GU disease in males. Urinary retention, difficulty urinating, and perineal and suprapubic pain are just a few of the symptoms of prostatitis.

Clinical symptoms of epididymitis include discomfort, scrotal and testicular edema, and, rarely, a draining sinus. Tubo-ovarian abscesses, endometritis, and salpingitis are all possible complications for female patients with GU system dissemination. A worsening of the situation may occur if the inflammation spreads to the peritoneum and omentum, with or without the emergence of ascites.

A man with Blastomyces prostatitis was able to infect his wife with endometrial cancer after the two of them had sexual contact. Only this one case of sexual transmission has ever been documented.

# Central nervous system blastomycosis (CNS)

Central nervous system blastomycosis is not likely to affect more than 5–10% of immunocompetent people. Infection in the CNS, as manifested by meningitis, epidural abscess, or brain abscess, can result from either hematogenous seeding or direct penetration through untreated skull-base osteomyelitis.

**Symptoms may include:**

Headaches,

Focal neurologic abnormalities,

Disorientation,

Alterations in vision,

Seizures.

Meningitis patients exhibit elevated protein levels and hypoglycemia in their cerebrospinal fluid (CSF), in addition to lymphocytic or neutrophilic pleocytosis.

About 45 percent of the time, Blastomyces will grow in CSF cultures; nevertheless, a positive CSF Blastomyces antigen may facilitate diagnosis. Some of the CNS issues that have been described include hydrocephalus, edematous mass effect, cerebral herniation, infarction, seizures, panhypopituitarism, paralysis, and poor academic performance.

## Pathogenesis

The Phenomenal Phase Shifts

The ability of dimorphic fungi, like Blastomyces spp., to change their morphology from mold to yeast is crucial to comprehending their pathogenicity.

The temperature change has a crucial role in this morphological change or phase transition. It is an intricate procedure that calls for systemic alterations in transcription, metabolism, cellular signaling, cell wall composition, and lipid content of the plasma membrane. These two shifts take place at the same time.

The conidia-producing molds B. dermatitidis and B. Gilchrist thrive at soil temperatures of 22-25 degrees Celsius (spores). Aerosolized conidia and mold pieces inhaled into the lungs of a human host at 37 degrees Celsius after the soil has been disturbed, often as a result of human activity, transform into pathogenic yeast. The immune system of the host can be fooled by this yeast, allowing it to spread infection.

Yeast can more easily develop from conidia that have been ingested by lung macrophages. Not only do Blastomyces prefer an intracellular lifestyle, but so do other dimorphic pathogens like H. capsulatum, Coccidioides spp., and Paracoccidioides spp. Unlike other fungi, such as H. capsulatum and Cryptococcus neoformans, B. dermatitidis may not use the "Trojan Horse" strategy of macrophage survival to spread extrapulmonary.

Researchers have been able to pinpoint genes necessary for the yeast-to-fungus phase transition and pathogenicity thanks to the advent of molecular techniques that enable the genetic manipulation of dimorphic fungi.

Both DRK1 (dimorphism-regulating kinase-1) and BAD1 (beta-amyloid deficient-1) are examples of such genes (Blastomyces adhesion-1; formerly WI-1).

Fungi such as B. dermatitidis, B. Gilchrist, and H. capsulatum undergo a metamorphosis from mold to yeast when exposed to higher

---

temperatures (between 22 and 37 degrees Celsius).

This transformation requires a hybrid histidine kinase, which is encoded by the DRK1 gene. 27 Cells of Blastomyces and Histoplasma that have had their DRK1 gene removed grow as hyphae instead of yeast when cultured at 37 degrees Celsius.

DRK1 null mutants (DRK1) fail to express BAD1, a key virulence factor, and also have an abnormal distribution of cell wall polysaccharides such as -(1,3)-glucan and chitin. In a mouse model of lung infection, Blastomyces and Histoplasma cells with reduced transcription of DRK-1 are not pathogenic, meaning they do not cause disease. These findings provide genetic support that the transition from bacteria to yeast is necessary for pathogenicity.

B. dermatitidis expresses BAD1, a protein with a 120-kDa molecular weight that helps with adhesion and immune evasion, during the yeast phase of its life cycle. BAD1 is a protein that is produced by B. dermatitidis yeast and then secreted into the extracellular milieu. It then interacts with chitin found in the cell wall to bind back to the cell surface.

BAD1 is an adhesin that binds heparan sulfate and performs the role of attaching yeast cells to the tissue of the host.

Repressing the production of TNF- by BAD1 makes immune evasion possible. This is accomplished in a manner that is both dependent and independent of transforming growth factor- (TGF-). 30 TNF- is an essential cytokine that contributes to the host's defense against an infection caused by Blastomyces.

When TNF- is neutralized in mice, a progressive form of pulmonary blastomycosis develops in the animals. In addition to the effects it has on the innate immune system, BAD1 also affects the adaptive immune system. It does this by inhibiting the activation of CD4+ T lymphocytes, which in turn decreases the production of interleukin-17 (IL-17) and interferon-gamma (INF-).

The BAD1 null mutants (BAD1) strains are avirulent in a mouse model of lung infection but not in other murine models.

In addition, the lungs of mice that have been infected with BAD1 strains appear to be morphologically normal and contain a limited number of granulomas. In addition to BAD-1, other genes that are upregulated during pulmonary infection have been identified by in vivo transcriptional profiling of B. dermatitidis yeast during pulmonary infection.

Changes in the cell wall carbohydrate content may potentially contribute to virulence and immune evasion as the fungus transitions from its yeast phase to its yeast phase. During the transformation from mold to yeast, the percentage of -(1,3)-glucan found in the cell wall rises, while the percentage of -(1,3)-glucan drops from 40–50% in mycelia to less than 5% in yeast.

This occurs because yeast has a more complex cell wall structure than mold does. It is impossible to use (1,3) -glucan assays for diagnosis, and echinocandins are rendered ineffective as a result of the decreased -(1,3)-glucan concentration in the cell walls of Blastomyces yeast.

These are just two of the significant diagnostic and therapeutic implications that result from this.

Alternately, the transition from yeast to mycelia is essential for environmental survival, mating to increase genetic diversity, and transmission to mammalian hosts. Yeast and mycelia are both essential components of fungi.

Current genetic research has led to the discovery of a GATA transcription factor that is encoded by SREB and is responsible for mediating the transition from yeast to mycelia following a temperature reduction from 37 to 22 degrees Celsius. 34 SREB null mutants (SREB) have a failure in the morphologic shift that correlates to a decrease in the manufacture of neutral lipids (ergosterol, triacylglycerol), as well as the development of lipid droplets.

At a temperature of 22 degrees Celsius, the N-acetylglucosamine transporters NGT1 and NGT2 in B. dermatitidis and H. capsulatum speed up the transition to mycelia.

# Host Reaction

It is necessary to have both an innate immune response and an adaptive immunological response to resist a Blastomyces infection, although humoral immunity is not required.

After inhalation of aerosolized conidia, alveolar macrophages, and neutrophils phagocytize and eliminate the fungal spores. However, conidia that make it through phagocytosis eventually germinate into yeast, which is a more difficult target for the immune system of the host to eliminate.

The yeast of B. dermatitidis actively undermines the immune defenses of the host by inhibiting the production of cytokines by host cells, impeding the activation of CD4+ T lymphocytes, and suppressing the production of nitric oxide.

In addition, Blastomyces yeast exhibits a reasonable amount of resistance to the reactive oxygen species that are generated by macrophages and neutrophils.

After recovering from blastomycosis, hosts establish cell-mediated immunity that lasts for at least two years38 and most likely for a longer period.

## Clinical Manifestations

The clinical manifestations of blastomycosis are diverse and can range from asymptomatic infection to pneumonia to acute respiratory distress syndrome.

Blastomycosis is a fungus that causes blastomycosis (ARDS). Blastomycosis has been given the nickname "the great impostor" because of the clinical heterogeneity that it exhibits. Following the disruption of the soil, aerosolized conidia most commonly enter the body through the lungs.

There have been reports of traumatic inoculations of the skin, such as those that occur in laboratories. Following the inhalation of mycelial pieces or spores, the onset of symptoms can take anywhere from three weeks to three and a half months. 4,41 Around 25–40% of patients who are already experiencing symptoms will develop extrapulmonary spread.

The skin, bones, genitourinary tract, and central nervous system (CNS) are common locations for disseminated disease; however, Blastomyces can infect nearly every organ in the body.

## Blastomycosis in Those Who Have Weak Immune Systems (HIV/AID, Women Who Are Pregnant and Their Newborn Babies)

### HIV/AIDS

In contrast to histoplasmosis, blastomycosis is a far less prevalent infection found in HIV/AIDS patients.

The majority of HIV patients who develop blastomycosis have a CD4+ T-lymphocyte count that is lower than 200 cells/mm3, and the majority of these individuals also have a history of having other opportunistic infections.

Patients with AIDS have an increased risk of developing severe lung disease (such as ARDS or miliary disease), and up to forty percent of these patients develop spread to the central nervous system.

In one case study, it was hypothesized that the reactivation of a dormant infection was responsible for approximately one-quarter of the cases of blastomycosis that were connected to AIDS.

Patients diagnosed with AIDS and blastomycosis had a mortality rate that exceeded fifty percent before the development of current antiretrovirals.

## The Transplantation of Solid Organs (SOT)

Among SOT recipients, blastomycosis is a relatively rare infection, with a cumulative frequency of 0.13 - 0.14% in patients who come from endemic areas.

This rate is significantly lower than the incidence of post-transplant coccidioidomycosis or histoplasmosis that has been recorded. After a transplant, the start of the illness can take anywhere from 12 days to 250 months to manifest itself. This diversity may be a reflection of diverse disease etiology, including initial infection, (ii) reactivation of latent disease, and (iii) the conversion of recently acquired, pre-transplant, asymptomatic infection into symptomatic disease. On the other hand, in contrast to histoplasmosis and

There have been no cases of coccidioidomycosis or donor-derived blastomycosis recorded. SOT patients exhibit similar rates of disseminated disease (33–50%) when compared to immunocompetent hosts, but they are at a greater risk for severe pulmonary disease including respiratory failure and ARDS.

The mortality rate for transplant-associated blastomycosis varies from 33–38%, but it jumps up to 67% in patients who also have ARDS.

If blastomycosis has been treated effectively, patients typically do not need to continue taking suppressive antifungal medication for the rest of their lives.

## Therapy with anti-TNF antibodies

When it comes to the host's immune response against blastomycosis, TNF- is an extremely important cytokine. In murine models, the progression of lung infection is seen when TNF- is neutralized by antibodies that are antibody-mediated.

Case reports are the only source of clinical data about blastomycosis in the context of TNF- exposure; there is very little of it.

Notwithstanding this, blastomycosis was included in the warning that the Food and Drug Administration published in 2008 about the increased risk of fulminant infections with endemic mycosis in patients who were getting TNF inhibitor therapy.

## Blastomycosis in Women Who Are Pregnant and Their Newborn Babies

Blastomycosis in pregnant women and newborns is extremely uncommon, and clinical knowledge is based almost entirely on case reports.

It does not matter which trimester a woman is in when she becomes infected with the disease; nevertheless, the condition is most commonly diagnosed in the second or third trimester.

According to case reports, disseminated disease accounts for 62% of cases, while isolated pulmonary infections only account for 38%.

Placental involvement has been recorded, however, there is a lack of reliable data regarding the frequency of placental infection because testing by culture or histology has been conducted in only one-third of clinical cases.

Blastomycosis does not appear to raise the risk for congenital abnormalities; nonetheless, there is the possibility that the infection could be passed on during the peripartum period.

Rare but potentially dangerous, neonatal pulmonary blastomycosis affects an infant's lungs.

There is a lack of clarity about the underlying etiology of newborn blastomycosis, which may entail transplacental transfer or the aspiration of contaminated vaginal secretions.

Individuals with healthy immune systems can contract this virus. Blastomycosis is an opportunistic illness that is less prevalent than histoplasmosis or coccidioidomycosis but can be more severe in immunocompromised patients. It's more common to contract coccidioidomycosis or histoplasmosis.

At room temperature, B. dermatitidis-containing mold thrives in soil fertilized with animal feces and in wet, rotting, acidic organic matter.

Locations close to rivers often have these characteristics.

When breathed, spores develop into 15-20 micrometer-sized yeasts that can cause serious infections. Yeasts of this type produce distinctively broad-based buds.

The virus may have spread to the lungs, which for the time being, keeps it in your lungs.

## Hematogenous dissemination

The skin, prostate, epididymides, testes, seminal vesicles, kidneys, vertebrae, ends of long bones, subcutaneous tissues, central nervous system, oral or nasal mucosa, thyroid, lymph nodes, and bone marrow are just a few of the organs that might get infected after hematogenous dissemination. Systemic infections can also be caused by hematogenous spread.

# Signs and Symptoms of Blastomycosis

## Pulmonary

Sometimes there are no symptoms at all, and pulmonary blastomycosis is misdiagnosed as an acute illness that goes away on its own. It can also begin mildly before progressing into a chronic infection with increasing severity. Some of the symptoms include a dry or productive hacking cough, chest pain, shortness of breath, high temperature, shivers, and profuse perspiring.

Pleural effusion can occur on occasion. Acute respiratory distress syndrome can develop quickly during the course of some infections, making breathing difficult for the patient.

## *Extrapulmonary*

The signs and symptoms of extrapulmonary disseminated blastomycosis shift from organ to organ.

The vast majority of cases of disease spread manifest as skin lesions, which may be singular or multiple and may or may not be accompanied by overt lung involvement. Sometimes pulmonary involvement occurs alongside skin lesions. Papules, often called papulopustular, are little bumps that develop in sunlight.

Asymptomatic abscesses with pinprick to one-millimeter diameters occur on the widening margins of the lesion. Papillae, which look like warts, can sometimes grow in an asymmetrical pattern on surfaces. Sometimes bumps called bullae appear.

Eventually, the lesions' cores will heal, but the lesions themselves will continue to expand, leaving behind atrophic scars. After each lesion has fully matured, it appears as a raised verrucous patch with a purple-red, abscess-studded border and a width of less than two millimeters. When germs form a superinfection, ulceration might occur.

Bone lesions can cause the skin above the affected area to swell, become painfully hot, and cause significant discomfort.

Genital lesions can cause a variety of symptoms, including an enlarged epididymis, acute pain in the perineum, or tenderness in the prostate detected during a rectal exam.

Infections of the central nervous system can cause a variety of symptoms, including:

Brain abscess,

Epidural abscess

Meningitis.

# CHAPTER 3
# BLASTOMYCOSIS
# SKIN(CUTANEOUS PAPULOPUSTULAR)

The skin is the most prevalent extrapulmonary site of infection, and individuals with disseminated illness might have cutaneous involvement in anywhere from 40–80 percent of cases

## Papulopustular lesions

Are frequently the first sign of cutaneous disease, however, they can later advance to ulcerative, verrucous, or crusty lesions. Additional manifestations include violaceous nodules, plaques, and abscesses.

Erythema nodosum is frequently seen in individuals who have histoplasmosis or coccidioidomycosis, but it is only infrequently recorded in people who have an infection caused by Blastomyces.

## Cutaneous lesions

Have the potential to grow in an asymmetrical pattern, leading to the development of ulcerations and necrosis, both of which can result in deformity, including scarring that is permanent.

In a smaller percentage of cases, cutaneous blastomycosis will present itself as a draining sinus tract or ulcer caused by underlying osteomyelitis.

Lesions on the skin can appear everywhere on the body, although they most commonly appear on regions of the body that are exposed to the elements, such as the head and the extremities.

Blastomycosis is much less likely to involve the mucous membranes than H. capsulatum or Paracoccidioides spp., but intra-oral, nasal, and pharyngeal lesions have occasionally been described. Blastomycosis is caused by a fungus called Blastomyces.

The cutaneous involvement of the eyelid is the most prevalent discovery in ophthalmology, even though it is unusual. Endophthalmitis and orbital abscesses are two conditions that are quite uncommon.

Ectropion, which can be worsened by the involvement of the periorbital skin and may require surgical correction following successfully treating an infection can complicate matters.

Skin lesions on the face, neck, and extremities are common when the infection spreads from the lungs to the rest of the body. A lesion, or several lesions, could appear.

Papules, pustules, and subcutaneous nodules are the starting points for most lesions.

Eventually, the lesions will develop into ulcers and lead to crusty sores.

After a few months to a year or more of healing, a lesion will leave a raised scar that looks like a wart. Extreme disfigurement may occur if lesions spread over a wide area of the face.

Permanent scarring is a common complication.

A lesion of the skin caused by blastomycosis

Symptoms of infection with the fungus Blastomyces dermatitidis include the development of a skin lesion known as blastomycosis.

When the fungus travels throughout the body, it causes an infection to develop on the skin. There is also a variety of blastomycosis that affects only the skin and, in most cases, improves on its own over time. This page addresses the more pervasive variety of the virus.

## Causes:

The fungal infection known as blastomycosis is extremely uncommon. It is most frequently observed in:

Africa

Canada's south-central and north-central regions, as well as the region around the Great Lakes States of America

India

Israel

Saudi Arabia

A person can become infected with the fungus if they breathe in spores that are present in damp soil, particularly in areas where there is decomposing plant matter.

This virus poses a greater threat to those whose immune systems are compromised, but even healthy people are not immune to the possibility of contracting this disease.

The fungus attacks the lungs after it has entered the body through the respiratory system. When this happens, the fungus is said to have "disseminated" to other parts of the body of the affected individual.

This infection may affect a variety of systems, including the skin, bones, and joints, as well as the genitals and urinary tract. Skin signs are an indication that blastomycosis has diffused throughout the body.

Lesions on the skin can appear everywhere on the body, although they most commonly appear on regions of the body that are exposed to the elements, such as the head and the extremities.

---

The cutaneous involvement of the eyelid is the most prevalent discovery in ophthalmology, even though it is unusual. Endophthalmitis and orbital abscesses are two conditions that are quite uncommon.

Ectropion, which can be worsened by the involvement of the periorbital skin and may require surgical correction following successful treatment of infection, can make the situation more difficult.

As the infection moves from the lungs to other areas of the body, it frequently causes lesions of the skin to appear on the face, the neck, and the limbs. One or more lesions may develop.

Lesions originate as papules, pustules, or as subcutaneous nodules.

In a matter of weeks or months, the lesions will transform into ulcers and produce crusty sores.

Lesions can take anywhere from a few months to a few years to fully heal, at which point they become elevated scars that resemble warts. Lesions can spread across a large portion of the face, which can result in serious deformity.

# CHAPTER 4
# BLASTOMYCOSIS IN DOGS

Blastomycosis is a fungal infection that is caused in dogs by fungi belonging to the Blastomyces genus.

Dogs frequently suffer from the fungal condition known as blastomycosis. People can catch the infection in the same way as dogs do. There is no transmission of disease from one animal to another.

And does not spread to other people. Infections of blastomycosis in other species, such as cats, are extremely uncommon.

## Manifestations and Methods of Diagnosis

Diseases of the respiratory system are common. Congestion, chest tightness, and coughing are some of the symptoms of this illness. Blastomycosis is a fungal infection that can affect many other parts of the body, including the eyes, the skin, the bones, and the lymph nodes.

If blastomycosis is detected, a veterinary professional will need to carry out a comprehensive physical examination. This will involve looking in the mouth, inspecting all regions of the skin, looking in the eyes, and using a stethoscope to listen to the heart and lungs.

Because blastomycosis is so frequently seen in the lungs, it is usual practice to take X-rays of the chest.

Blood tests and urine testing can be used to detect organ dysfunction and sometimes for diagnosis; however, the majority of cases of blastomycosis can only be diagnosed through the microscopic inspection of parts of the affected tissues.

## Breeds That Are Affected

Blastomycosis is a disease that can affect any kind of dog. It appears that large-breed dogs are more likely to contract the disease.

This could be because large breed dogs, as opposed to small breed dogs, are utilized more frequently for activities such as hunting and working in environments with a higher prevalence of Blastomyces fungus, such as forests.

Dogs of any age or gender can become afflicted with the disease.

## Treatment

Antifungal drugs used over an extended period are required for the treatment of blastomycosis. Itraconazole or fluconazole is the antifungal agent that is utilized most frequently. It may be necessary to first hospitalize some dogs to assist with the management of some of their more severe symptoms. Some dogs will respond to treatment, but then they will acquire symptoms once again after they stop taking the antifungals.

There is a possibility that some of the initial symptoms, such as blindness, will not go away. If the animal is responsive to treatment, the prognosis—that is, the likelihood that it will survive with a high quality of life—is extremely favorable.

To successfully treat this disease in dogs, treatment may need to be administered for several months (at least four to six months in most cases). In certain circumstances, the medicine amphotericin B, ketoconazole, or a combination of the two may be prescribed.

## *What is the outlook for my dog's condition?*

In many instances of blastomycosis infection, the prognosis is favorable, with recovery rates ranging between 50 and 75%.

There is no way to determine this before the treatment has begun; nonetheless, the chances of survival are lower for a dog that is in poor condition or has an advanced stage of the disease.

When the medicine begins to take effect and the fungus begins to die off, many people find that the first twenty-four to seventy-two hours are the most important.

As a rule, the lungs are home to a significant number of these fungal species; hence, a severe inflammatory reaction may take place, leading to difficulty breathing or even respiratory collapse.

Although chest X-rays are not always able to accurately anticipate the result of treatment, your veterinarian will take radiographs (x-rays) of your dog's chest before treatment to evaluate the state of the lungs.

When the fungus invades the neurological system, the testicles, or the eyes, relapses of blastomycosis are typically more likely. Because many medications have trouble penetrating the natural protective barriers of various biological systems, it is considerably more challenging to get rid of organisms that are located in these areas.

Castration of male canines may be required to get rid of this possible source of organisms. A similar procedure may be performed to remove one or both of the animal's eyes, especially if the condition has already caused the animal to become blind.

Even in cases when it would appear that therapy was successful, there is still a very real possibility of relapse with this illness. Regular checkups in the form of physical examinations, radiography, and laboratory tests are part of the follow-up testing.

It is generally recommended to evaluate the success of treatment using the MiraVista urine antigen test to decide when it is safe to stop taking medication and to identify whether or not treatment was successful.

## Is it possible that my pet could give me an infection?

According to research conducted on the fungus, once an animal is infected with it, the organism transforms into another form or phase that does not appear to be contagious to other animals or humans.

When dealing with any draining lesions, however, proper hygiene must be adhered to at all times. This is just good sense. After coming into contact with an infected animal, people who work with animals should always wash their hands properly and wear gloves designed for protection.

In the majority of instances, it is not necessary to quarantine the diseased pet from the other members of the family, including humans and other animals.

Sharing the same environment as the person who contracted the illness in the first place probably poses the greatest threat of spreading it to other people (i.e., soil).

You must discuss the diagnosis of your pet with your family doctor because the Blastomyces bacterium may be found in the environment surrounding your home.

## The Expense of Veterinary Care

The diagnosis and treatment of blastomycosis can run a patient a significant amount of money. The costs of laboratory studies, x-rays, and biopsies might range anywhere from $500 to $1500.

Antifungal medication taken for an extended time can also be rather pricey. The price per month could range anywhere from $150 to $750, depending on the size of the dog and the dosage.

## Prevention

At this time, there is no vaccination available to protect against blastomycosis. To reduce the risk of developing a severe illness, it is critical to undergo timely examinations and receive appropriate medical care as soon as possible.

# CHAPTER 5

# THE BLASTOMYCES DERMATITIDIS BACTERIUM

At room temperature, Blastomyces dermatitidis thrives as a mycelial fungus, but when the temperature is raised to 37 degrees Celsius, it transforms into yeast.

Although these organisms have not been thoroughly researched, they occur naturally in the warm, wet soil of woodland areas that are also abundant in organic detritus.

Outdoorsmen and hunters have an increased risk of contracting B. dermatitidis. It is believed that it enters the lung, which then results in the production of a widespread pyogranulomatous infection through hematogenous dissemination including the lungs, skin, bone, and genitourinary system. Endophthalmitis brought on by this factor is not particularly common. Amphotericin is the drug of choice for therapy.

# Infection caused by fungi in the recipient of an organ transplant

## *Blastomycosis*

A mold of the type Blastomyces dermatitidis can be seen growing on rotting wood. These organisms have a distribution pattern that is geographically comparable to that of H. capsulatum (the midwest and southeastern United States).

Infection in humans can occur following the inhalation of aerosols that are loaded with conidia. In terms of clinical presentation, pulmonary symptoms such as coughing, spitting up mucus, chest pain, and shortness of breath are most prominent.

Radiological abnormalities include hilar adenopathy and infiltrates that are not specific to the disease. It is not uncommon for a disseminated infection to result in the involvement of metastatic skin, which manifests as massive nodular skin lesions that subsequently necrotize and fibrosis.

Infections in the genitourinary system and the skeletal system are two more common sources of metastatic dissemination.

Blastomycosis is one of the systemic mycoses that can infect a transplant recipient, however, it is one of the less prevalent types.

In most cases, a biopsy is required for diagnosis to perform the necessary histopathologic and cultural analyses. The first step in treatment is typically the intravenous administration of an amphotericin preparation, followed by the administration of itraconazole orally.

The function of contemporary antifungals is continuously being investigated and defined.

## Pulmonary Illness and Its Molecular Foundations

### *Blastomyces dermatitidis*

Blastomyces dermatitidis is another endemic species that can only be found in the middle of the United States, specifically in the Ohio River basin and the Mississippi River valley. Campers and other people who spend time outside are putting themselves in danger because it is typically present in forested areas during the rainy seasons.

*The clinical manifestations of the disease include:*

A cutaneous form and

A systemic type

With the latter starting in the lungs after being breathed in. Fever, general malaise, and chest pain are the nonspecific symptoms associated with an acute lung infection.

Imaging examinations might reveal infiltrates or something that looks like a mass of infiltrates.

As a result, the diagnosis of a Blastomyces infection may be delayed since the illness might mimic other disorders.

Some patients develop chronic disease with cavitation or progressive pulmonary blastomycosis, which manifests as acute respiratory distress syndrome, cavitary lesions, and a poor prognosis.

Other patients do not develop chronic disease but do develop progressive pulmonary blastomycosis.

The pathogenesis of a Blastomyces infection is comparable to that of histoplasmosis, which is characterized by necrotizing granulomas.

On the other hand, the lesions are significantly larger and have a greater amount of neutrophil necrosis. In addition, the organisms range in size from 8 to 15 microns and have obvious broad-based budding. They are visible when stained with hematoxylin and eosin according to standard procedures.

## Infectious Disorders of the Kidney

The fungus known as Blastomyces dermatitidis is the one that causes blastomycosis. Inhalation is the primary mode of transmission for the budding yeast B. dermatitidis, which is most commonly found in the soil.

The eastern United States, Canada, and certain areas of Africa are the only places in which the fungus may be found naturally.

Even while pulmonary blastomycosis accounts for the great majority of symptomatic cases, disseminated illness can develop in immunocompromised patients, and renal involvement can occur in up to ten percent of these instances.

The incidence of the disease is not considerably increased among immunosuppressed patients compared to that of the general population; nevertheless, the severity of the disease may be worse.

Individuals who have renal involvement will experience signs of pyelonephritis, such as discomfort in the flank, fever, and hematuria. Infections can cause renal abscesses and can spread through the renal capsule to cause perinephric abscesses.

Renal abscesses and perinephric abscesses are both types of abscesses.

---

**Granulomatous inflammation** and **significant acute inflammation** are both potential pathological characteristics that may be present. When stained with GMS, fungal organisms most typically take the form of broad-based budding yeast that ranges in diameter from 8 to 15 micrometers.

When compared to other types of yeast, such as H. capsulatum or Cryptococcus neoformans, B. dermatitidis can be distinguished from these other species due to its larger size and broad-based budding.

## Endemic mycoses

### Epidemiology

Blastomyces dermatitidis can be found in sporadic locations across Europe, Asia, Latin America, and Africa. In the United States, it is most commonly found along the river estuaries stretching from Minnesota to Mississippi.

In Canada, it can be found in the provinces bordering the Great Lakes. There are areas of warm, moist, sandy, acidic soil that are located in wooded areas that are rich in organic debris, at low elevations, and near bodies of water. These hyperendemic foci are found within the endemic area of the disease.

Although blastomycosis is typically linked to rural areas, urban foci of the disease have recently been reported. These urban foci of the disease have also been found near waterways. There is some overlap between the regions where blastomycosis and histoplasmosis are considered to be endemic.

There has been a correlation between outbreaks of illness and either occupational or recreational soil exposure. It is possible for outbreaks to involve patients of any age and of either gender; however, instances most frequently affect individuals in their early to middle twenties, and they are more frequently documented in males than in women.

Both diabetes and African-American race are factors that increase the likelihood of symptomatic conditions. Dogs have an extremely high risk of contracting blastomycosis and have the potential to serve as sentinels in point-source outbreaks.

## Infections of the Central Nervous System Caused by Yeasts and Molds

The Blastomyces Dermatitidis bacterium
In addition to its native habitat in Africa, the dimorphic fungus Blastomyces dermatitidis can also be found in specific regions of the lower Mississippi River Valley, the North Central

states, and the mid-Atlantic states of the continental United States.

It is generally accepted that spores are breathed in from a source located in the soil; however, the natural position of this organism in the environment has only been pinpointed sporadically.

The majority of people have a subclinical form of the disease, and rare cases of transmission have been observed.

Lesions of the lung, bone, and skin that are granulomatous and suppurating are some of the telltale signs of disseminated blastomycosis. It has been observed that blastomycosis can involve the brain in anywhere from 6 to 33 percent of cases when it has spread throughout the body.

Meningitis may be the first symptom that a patient with CNS blastomycosis has, even though individuals with this condition typically present with evidence of infection at other sites.

Blastomycosis meningitis is characterized by a chronic neutrophilic pleocytosis, which is a condition that only occurs seldom when CSF cultures are positive.

CNS involvement can sometimes be identified by the presence of a mass lesion (also known as blastomycosis) in the brain parenchyma.

Patients with compromised immune systems have an increased likelihood of becoming infected with B. dermatitidis.

Within a diverse population of immunocompromised patients, a review of 24 cases of infection with B. dermatitidis found 6 cases of disseminated disease, including 4 cases with involvement of the central nervous system (CNS).

# Diseases Caused by Mycobacteria, Fungi, Spirochetal Organisms, and Parasites

## Blastomycosis

The dimorphic fungus Blastomyces dermatitidis is endemic to the United States, occurring from the southeastern coast to the upper Midwest. Inhalation causes primary infection to occur in the lungs, much like it does with other types of soil fungi.

Lesions that are suppurative and granulomatous can be caused by a disseminated infection in some different places, including the lung, the skin, the bone, and the central nervous system.

The latter can be infected as frequently as one-third of the time, and the vast majority of individuals diagnosed with central nervous system blastomycosis show evidence of infection at other sites. Immune insufficiency, in contrast to many other fungal infections, does not appear to be a definite predisposing factor for the spread of the infection. Meningitis is the hallmark of the central nervous system (CNS) invasion, although some individuals go on to develop blastomycosis (focal abscesses).

In cases with blastomycosis meningitis, the cerebrospinal fluid (CSF) has been found to have a pleocytosis, with either a lymphocyte or neutrophil preponderance, in addition to high amounts of protein and low levels of glucose.

It is common knowledge that cultures are notoriously untrustworthy and almost always destructive. CSF that has been directly observed by a microscope may sometimes reveal the presence of the fungus, although smears are typically of no use.

When the cerebrospinal fluid (CSF) is extracted from the ventricles or cisterns,

---

certain authors claim a higher rate of positive culture results. Even if updated serological tests are in the process of being developed, the only way to establish a clear diagnosis is still through isolating the pathogen.

Pathologic conditions of the hypopharynx, larynx, and trachea that are not squamous

Blastomyces dermatitidis, also known as North American blastomycosis, Gilchrist's illness, and Chicago disease, is a fungus that is native to the Great Lakes region, as well as the basins of the Ohio and Mississippi rivers.

There have been reports of outbreaks of a minor nature in the states of North Carolina, Minnesota, Illinois, Wisconsin, and Kentucky, respectively.

Despite its name, it is not exclusive to North America; in fact, it has been found in South America and Africa as well. Passionate bird hunters run the risk of being injured or killed for reasons that will be explained later.

In the United States, the geographic distribution of canine blastomycosis is the same as that of the disease in humans. It has been observed that hunting dogs are particularly susceptible to developing blastomycosis.

A patient's history of having a pet dog that passed away due to a fungal disease can serve as a diagnostic indicator. Blastomycosis cannot be passed from humans to dogs unless by bites from infected dogs.

On occasion, Blastomyces have been isolated from soil specimens, particularly those that were found close to water. As is the case with other types of fungus, the only forms of yeast that may spread the infection are the arthrospores.

Point sources are typically found in locations that are heavily forested and have a significant amount of water, such as those that have been tracked to beaver ponds or building sites located in lakeside.

The incidence of infection is affected by a person's proximity to arthrospores; people who pick things up off the ground to study them are more likely to become infected with the fungus than those who examine things from a greater distance.

This would also explain the relationship of blastomycosis with bird hunters since they hide in wait for their prey by crouching or lying on the ground, as well as with their hunting dogs, which scent the ground.

Blastomyces have the potential to cause disease when it is breathed in, or when it is traumatically introduced into the skin.

It may present with an acute onset of fever, productive cough, and myalgias, or it may present with an insidious onset of weight loss, malaise, anorexia, and a chronic cough, mimicking tuberculosis. In either case, the symptoms may be difficult to diagnose.

Direct inoculation into soft tissues or the upper airway causes only local indicators, like an ulcerating mass, and no systemic symptoms in the infected person.

In 25% of individuals, an immunosuppressive state comes first, which is followed by fungal disease. Diabetes mellitus is another condition that is frequently linked to blastomycosis.

It would indicate that this organism has its sights set specifically on the larynx. A recent investigation conducted at the Mayo Clinic on 102 individuals diagnosed with blastomycosis found that five of those patients had laryngeal lesions.

An erythematous or white mass with irregular borders can be seen in patients who have laryngeal blastomycosis. This appearance, which is similar to that of carcinoma, can cause the vocal cords to become immobile.

There is a potential for the development of deep laryngeal fissures or pharynx cutaneous fistulas. Following the reporting of quite a few cases of laryngeal carcinoma, a second look at the tissues obtained from the biopsy or laryngectomy indicated blastomycosis rather than cancer in those patients.

## Fungal infections that have spread via the bloodstream hematogenous

The Blastomyces dermatitidis bacterium
The dimorphic fungus known as Blastomyces dermatitidis can be found in soil and rotting wood in the south-central and north-central regions of the United States and Canada, as

well as in certain regions of southern Europe and Africa.

In most cases, infection is brought on by breathing in infectious conidia, while inoculation is only occasionally responsible. The spectrum of symptoms includes asymptomatic infection up to severe involvement in multiple organ systems including ARDS.

The most common manifestation seen in clinical settings is an infection of the lungs, which can show as either acute or persistent pneumonia. Both acute and chronic forms of pneumonia can present with non-specific symptoms such as fever, chills, loss of weight, and a cough that produces purulent sputum.

Acute pneumonia is more likely to be confused with bacterial or viral pneumonia.

The skin is the most prevalent extrapulmonary location, and it typically displays lesions that are either verrucous, papular, or ulcerative. Blastomycosis can manifest itself in different ways, including osteomyelitis, prostatitis, epididymo orchitis, and meningitis.

Patients with a weakened immune system are more likely to suffer from a severe, multiorgan system disease associated with a high mortality rate.

These patients almost always have pulmonary findings, which may include diffuse interstitial or alveolar changes, ARDS, or respiratory failure.

These findings can also be a combination of these conditions. Lesions of the skin that are verrucous or ulcerative can be detected in persons who have this condition.

Blastomycosis is regarded as a consequence of advanced AIDS and typically affects patients whose CD4 counts are lower than 200.

Moreover, patients undergoing cytotoxic chemotherapy and corticosteroid therapy, as well as transplant recipients, have been shown to exhibit this condition.

Blastomycosis is relatively uncommon in pregnant women; nonetheless, there have been reports of perinatal transmission of the infection to neonates, which led to serious infections in infants.

Children are far more rarely affected by disease than adults are, yet the signs and symptoms of infection in children are very similar to those seen in immunocompetent adults.

Blastomycosis can be difficult to diagnose since it can look like other diseases, such as lung cancer, skin cancer, tuberculosis, histoplasmosis, nocardiosis, sarcoidosis, and others that fall under the category of granulomatous illnesses.

The infection may show up as a nodule, cavitary lesion, mass lesion, lobar consolidation, atypical pneumonia, diffuse interstitial illness, or military disease on the chest roentgenogram. On close inspection of tissue, sputum, bronchial washings, pleural fluid, pus, or urine sediment,

it is sometimes possible to see organisms in their natural state. Large, thick-walled, broad-based budding yeast forms are characteristic of the dermatitidis strain of B. dermatitidis.

It can take as long as four weeks for the culture to produce sufficient growth for identification, which can then be verified with a DNA probe.

An EIA for B. dermatitidis A antigen, a complement fixation assay, and an immunodiffusion assay are all available; however, none of them are sensitive enough or specific enough to be useful.

A novel assay for detecting Blastomyces antigen is most sensitive when performed on urine, although it can also be done on serum and cerebrospinal fluid. The test is not specific because it reacts with antigens from other organisms such as Histoplasma, Paracoccidioides, and Penicillium.

# CONCLUSION

The diagnosis and treatment of blastomycosis are not always easy to accomplish. Even in regions where blastomycosis is common, the disease's non-specific clinical symptoms usually cause a diagnosis to be made much later than it should be.

Certain clinical characteristics, such as persistent pneumonia despite appropriate management for CAP; (ii) simultaneous pulmonary and cutaneous infection; (iii) ARDS; and (iv) illness following recognizable risk factors for Blastomyces exposure, should raise suspicion among physicians practicing in areas where Blastomyces is endemic.

It is necessary to be aware of the fact that Blastomyces spp. are capable of infecting and spreading in immunocompetent as well as immunocompromised individuals. After gaining an awareness of phase transition, doctors will be reminded that -(1,3)-glucan tests and echinocandin antifungals do not play a role in the diagnosis or treatment of blastomycosis. And ultimately, a better understanding of the typical challenges faced by clinicians who prescribe polyene and azole antifungals would lead to a reduction in the hazards associated with treatment.

www.ingramcontent.com/pod-product-compliance
Lightning Source LLC
Chambersburg PA
CBHW051819250726
48659CB00005B/1572